I0696779

Isotonic Exercise for Beginners

Importance of Isotonic Exercise

By

Darroch Paxton

Copyright@2023

Table of Contents

CHAPTER 1
Introduction

1.1 Definition of Isotonic Exercise

Isotonic exercise is a form of physical activity that involves muscle contractions in which the length of the muscle changes while it generates a constant force to move a joint through a range of motion. In simpler terms, during isotonic exercise, the muscle shortens and lengthens while the tension remains relatively constant. This type of exercise is characterized by dynamic movements and is commonly associated with activities like weightlifting, resistance training, and traditional strength training exercises.

In isotonic exercises, muscles work against a resistance or load, which can be provided by various means such as dumbbells, barbells, resistance bands, or one's body weight. The constant tension on the muscle during these exercises makes them highly effective for building and toning muscle, increasing strength, and enhancing overall physical fitness. The dynamic nature of isotonic exercise also makes it a versatile choice for targeting different muscle groups and achieving various fitness goals.

1.2 Importance of Isotonic Exercise

The importance of isotonic exercise in maintaining and improving physical health cannot be overstated. This form of exercise offers a wide range of benefits, which include:

1. **Muscle Strength and Endurance:** Isotonic exercise is one of the most effective methods for increasing muscle strength and endurance. It stimulates muscle fibers to adapt and grow, leading to enhanced functional strength, improved performance in daily activities, and a reduced risk of injuries.

2. **Weight Management:** Isotonic exercise is integral to weight management and body composition. It helps burn calories and build lean muscle mass, which, in turn, increases metabolic rate. As muscle requires more energy at rest

than fat, it contributes to weight control and overall fitness.

3. **Flexibility and Range of Motion:** While isotonic exercise primarily focuses on strength, many isotonic movements involve a full range of motion. This enhances flexibility and joint mobility, reducing the risk of stiffness and musculoskeletal issues.

4. **Cardiovascular Health:** Some isotonic exercises can elevate heart rate and provide cardiovascular benefits. For instance, circuit training, which combines isotonic movements with brief periods of high-intensity aerobic exercises, promotes cardiovascular health while building muscle.

5. **Mental Well-being:** Engaging in isotonic exercise can have a positive impact on mental well-being. Physical activity triggers the release of endorphins, which can reduce stress, anxiety, and symptoms of depression, contributing to an improved overall quality of life.

6. **Bone Health:** Isotonic exercises, especially those involving resistance to gravity, like squats and lunges, can help maintain and improve bone density, reducing the risk of osteoporosis and fractures.

1.3 Historical Overview

The history of isotonic exercise is intertwined with the evolution of physical fitness and strength training.

Strength training has been a part of human history for centuries, dating back to ancient Greece and beyond. However, modern isotonic exercise methods and equipment have evolved significantly.

In the late 19th and early 20th centuries, pioneers in physical culture, like Eugen Sandow and George Hacken Schmidt, made significant contributions to strength training techniques. Sandow, often referred to as the "Father of Bodybuilding," promoted resistance exercise using various apparatuses and free weights. His performances showcased the aesthetic and functional benefits of isotonic exercise.

The 20th century saw the rise of weightlifting and bodybuilding as organized sports, with athletes like John Grimek and Steve Reeves becoming icons of strength and fitness. In the mid-20th century, the development of specialized weightlifting equipment and the introduction of standardized techniques solidified the place of isotonic exercise in fitness and sport.

Today, isotonic exercise has become a cornerstone of fitness and sports training. It has also found applications in physical rehabilitation and various therapeutic settings, emphasizing its role in promoting health, strength, and well-being across a wide spectrum of individuals and contexts.

CHAPTER 2

Types of Isotonic Exercises

2.1 Concentric Isotonic Exercise

Concentric isotonic exercises focus on the muscle shortening while generating force to move a joint through a range of motion. During the concentric phase, the muscle contracts and becomes shorter as it lifts a resistance. This phase is often considered the "lifting" or "positive" phase of an exercise. For example, when performing a bicep curl, the upward motion where you raise the dumbbell towards your shoulder is the concentric phase. Concentric exercises are crucial for building muscle strength and power. They are commonly used to target specific muscle groups and are an integral part of resistance training routines.

2.2 Eccentric Isotonic Exercise

Eccentric isotonic exercises, on the other hand, emphasize the lengthening of the muscle while under tension. This phase is often referred to as the "lowering" or "negative" phase of an exercise. Eccentric contractions are essential for muscle control, stability, and functional strength. They can create micro-tears in muscle fibers, stimulating muscle growth and repair. For example, in a bicep curl, the lowering of the dumbbell back to its starting position is the eccentric phase. Eccentric exercises are particularly beneficial for improving muscle endurance and reducing the risk of muscle imbalances and injuries.

2.3 Isotonic Exercise Equipment

Isotonic exercise can be performed using various types of equipment and tools, depending on individual preferences and fitness goals. Some common isotonic exercise equipment includes:

Free Weights: Dumbbells, barbells, and kettlebells are versatile tools for isotonic exercises. They allow for a wide range of movements and are effective for targeting specific muscle groups.

Resistance Bands: Resistance bands are portable and adaptable tools that provide varying levels of resistance. They are useful for adding resistance to isotonic exercises and can be used for both upper and lower body workouts.

Weight Machines: Gyms often feature weight machines that offer guided isotonic exercises for specific muscle groups. These machines are ideal for beginners and can help maintain proper form.

Body Weight: Many isotonic exercises can be performed using just your body weight, such as push-ups, squats, and lunges. These exercises are excellent for building strength and can be done anywhere.

Cable Machines: Cable machines come with adjustable pulleys and attachments that allow for a wide range of isotonic exercises. They provide constant tension throughout the movement.

Medicine Balls: Medicine balls are versatile for both strength and power exercises. They can be used for exercises like medicine ball slams and Russian twists.

Functional Training Equipment: Equipment like TRX suspension trainers and stability balls can be used for isotonic exercises that emphasize balance and core strength.

The choice of equipment often depends on your fitness goals, available resources, and personal preferences. Isotonic exercises can be customized to fit your needs, and the variety of equipment available ensures that you can create a well-rounded and effective workout routine to meet your fitness objectives.

CHAPTER 3

Benefits of Isotonic Exercise

3.1 Muscle Strength and Endurance

Isotonic exercise plays a significant role in improving muscle strength and endurance. Here are the benefits in more detail:

- **Increased Muscle Mass:** Isotonic exercises, especially those involving resistance or weight training, are highly effective in stimulating muscle growth. When you repeatedly challenge your muscles with resistance, they adapt by increasing in size and strength. This increased muscle mass contributes to improved overall strength and physical performance.

- **Enhanced Muscle Endurance:** Isotonic exercises, particularly when performed with higher repetitions and lower resistance, can help improve muscle endurance. This is beneficial for everyday activities and sports that require sustained effort. Endurance training can help delay the onset of muscle fatigue, allowing you to perform tasks or exercises for longer periods without feeling exhausted.

- **Functional Strength:** Isotonic exercises are known for developing functional strength, which is the ability to perform everyday tasks with ease. Whether it's lifting groceries, carrying a child, or maintaining proper posture, the strength gained through isotonic exercises translates into improved functionality in daily life.

- **Injury Prevention:** Building muscle strength and endurance can reduce the risk of injuries, especially in sports and physical activities. Strong muscles provide better joint stability and support, reducing the strain on tendons and ligaments. This can help prevent common injuries, such as sprains and strains.

3.2 Weight Management

Isotonic exercise is an essential component of weight management and body composition. Here are the benefits related to weight management:

- **Calorie Expenditure:** Isotonic exercises, especially those involving compound movements (working multiple muscle groups simultaneously), are effective at burning calories. The energy expended during these workouts contributes to a calorie deficit when combined with a balanced diet. This calorie deficit is crucial for weight loss or weight maintenance.

- **Lean Muscle Mass:** Isotonic exercises not only help burn calories but also build lean muscle mass. Muscle tissue is metabolically active, meaning it requires more energy to maintain than fat tissue. As you increase your muscle mass through isotonic exercise, your resting metabolic rate (the number of calories burned at rest) goes up, making it easier to maintain a healthy weight.

- **Improved Body Composition:** Isotonic exercise can lead to a positive shift in body composition. By reducing body fat percentage and increasing muscle mass, you achieve a more toned and defined appearance. This can boost self-esteem and body confidence.

- **Sustainable Weight Management:** Unlike crash

diets or extreme weight loss programs, isotonic exercise promotes sustainable weight management. It's a long-term approach to health and fitness that not only helps you lose weight but also maintain it over time.

- **Metabolic Health:** Regular isotonic exercise can improve metabolic health by enhancing insulin sensitivity and reducing the risk of metabolic conditions like type 2 diabetes. It also helps regulate blood sugar levels and control appetite.

Isotonic exercise offers a multitude of benefits, including increased muscle strength, endurance, and improved weight management. These advantages not only enhance physical performance but also contribute to overall health and well-being. Incorporating isotonic exercise into your fitness routine can help you achieve and maintain your fitness and weight-related goals.

3.3 Flexibility and Range of Motion

Isotonic exercise, while primarily known for building strength, also has a positive impact on flexibility and range of motion. Here are the benefits in more detail:

- **Improved Joint Flexibility:** Many isotonic exercises involve movements through a full range of motion. For example, squats and lunges require bending the hips and knees deeply. Over time, these exercises can increase joint flexibility, reducing the risk of stiffness and promoting overall joint health.

- **Enhanced Muscle Lengthening:** Isotonic exercises, particularly when incorporating eccentric contractions (lengthening of the muscle under tension), contribute to muscle lengthening. This can be especially beneficial for individuals who have tight or shortened muscles, helping them regain normal muscle length and function.

- **Reduced Risk of Injury:** Greater flexibility and range of motion help reduce the risk of injury. Well-stretched and flexible muscles and joints are less prone to strains, sprains, and other musculoskeletal injuries, both during exercise and in daily activities.

- **Enhanced Athletic Performance:** For athletes and sports enthusiasts, improved flexibility and range of motion are essential. It allows for better movement and agility, enabling athletes to perform at their best and reduce the risk of overuse injuries.

- **Pain Relief:** Isotonic exercises, especially those that emphasize stretching and lengthening, can provide relief from chronic conditions such as lower back pain, muscle tightness, and joint discomfort.

3.4 Cardiovascular Health

While isotonic exercises are primarily associated with building muscle, they can also have positive effects on cardiovascular health when performed in specific ways:

- **Increased Heart Rate:** Some isotonic exercises, particularly those performed at higher intensities with minimal rest between sets, can elevate heart rate and provide cardiovascular benefits. For example, circuit training, which combines isotonic movements with brief periods of high-intensity aerobic exercises like jumping jacks or burpees, can significantly increase cardiovascular fitness.

- **Calorie Burn:** Intense isotonic exercises that work multiple muscle groups simultaneously, such as compound movements, can result in a high calorie burn. This can contribute to weight loss and better cardiovascular health by reducing the risk factors associated with heart disease.

- **Lowering Blood Pressure:** Regular isotonic exercise can help lower blood pressure, reducing the risk of hypertension. It promotes better blood vessel function and can lead to improved circulation.

- **Cholesterol Management:** Isotonic exercise can positively affect cholesterol levels by increasing the levels of HDL (good) cholesterol and decreasing LDL (bad) cholesterol. This can lower the risk of atherosclerosis and heart disease.

- **Stress Reduction:** Exercise, including isotonic exercise, triggers the release of endorphins, which are natural mood boosters. Reduced stress and anxiety can have a positive impact on cardiovascular health, as chronic stress is associated with heart problems.

Isotonic exercise not only contributes to muscle strength but also enhances flexibility, range of motion, and cardiovascular health. These combined benefits make isotonic exercise a well-rounded approach to overall physical well-being and a key component of a healthy and balanced fitness routine.

CHAPTER 4

How to Perform Isotonic Exercises

4.1 Proper Form and Technique

Performing isotonic exercises with proper form and technique is crucial to maximize the benefits of the exercises and reduce the risk of injury. Here are some key considerations:

- **Warm-Up:** Always start with a proper warm-up. Spend 5-10 minutes engaging in light aerobic activity, such as jogging or jumping jacks, to increase blood flow to your muscles and prepare them for the upcoming exercises.

- **Maintain Proper Posture:** Ensure that your body is in the correct position throughout the exercise. Maintain a neutral spine, engage your core, and keep your shoulders relaxed. Proper posture is vital for preventing injuries and getting the most out of the exercise.

- **Full Range of Motion:** Perform isotonic exercises through their full range of motion. This helps improve flexibility and ensures that you're working the entire muscle group effectively.

- **Controlled Movements:** Move slowly and with control. Avoid using momentum to lift or lower weights, as this can lead to improper form and potential injury.

- **Breathing:** Remember to breathe consistently throughout the exercise. Typically, you exhale during the concentric phase (when lifting or pushing) and inhale during the eccentric phase (when lowering or returning to the starting position).

- **Proper Weight Selection:** Choose a weight or resistance level that challenges you but still allows you to complete the desired number of repetitions with good form. If you're struggling to maintain proper form, the weight may be too heavy.

- **Seek Guidance:** If you're new to isotonic exercise, consider working with a qualified fitness professional, such as a personal trainer. They can help you learn and practice proper form and technique.

4.2 Safety Considerations

Safety is paramount when performing isotonic exercises. Here are some safety considerations to keep in mind:

- **Consult Your Healthcare Provider:** If you have any medical conditions or concerns about your fitness level, consult with a healthcare provider before starting a new exercise routine.

- **Start Slowly:** If you're new to isotonic exercise, begin with lighter weights and gradually increase the intensity as you become more comfortable with the movements.

- **Use Proper Equipment:** Ensure that any equipment you use is in good condition and set up correctly. Check for loose parts or frayed resistance bands.

- **Avoid Overtraining:** Give your muscles time to recover. Overtraining can lead to fatigue and injuries. It's recommended to allow 48 hours of rest for a muscle group before working it again.

- **Stay Hydrated:** Proper hydration is essential for overall health and safety during exercise. Drink water before, during, and after your workout.

- **Listen to Your Body:** If you experience pain, dizziness, shortness of breath, or any unusual symptoms during exercise, stop immediately and seek medical attention if necessary.

- **Use Spotters:** When lifting heavy weights, especially with barbells, use a spotter to assist and ensure safety.

4.3 Creating a Workout Routine

To incorporate isotonic exercises into a balanced workout routine, follow these steps:

- **Set Clear Goals:** Determine your fitness goals, whether they involve building strength, improving endurance, or increasing muscle mass.

- **Choose Exercises:** Select isotonic exercises that align with your goals. Include a mix of compound movements (exercises that work multiple muscle groups) and isolation exercises (targeting specific muscles).

- **Frequency:** Aim to perform isotonic exercises 2-4 times a week, allowing for muscle recovery between sessions.

- **Repetitions and Sets:** Depending on your goals, perform 2-5 sets of 8-15 repetitions for each exercise.

Adjust the weight or resistance accordingly.

- **Progression:** As you become stronger, gradually increase the weight or resistance level to continue challenging your muscles.

- **Rest Periods:** Allow 30-60 seconds of rest between sets, and 48 hours of rest for a specific muscle group before working it again.

- **Cool Down:** Finish your workout with a cool-down period that involves stretching and deep breathing exercises to promote muscle recovery and flexibility.

- **Variety:** Keep your routine fresh by varying exercises and adding new ones over time to prevent plateaus and boredom.

By following these guidelines, you can create a safe and effective isotonic exercise routine tailored to your fitness goals and needs. Always remember to prioritize safety and proper technique to ensure a successful and injury-free workout.

CHAPTER 5

Examples of Isotonic Exercises

5.1 Isotonic Exercises for Upper Body

1. Bicep Curl:

- Stand with a dumbbell in each hand, arms fully extended.

- Keeping your upper arms stationary, bend your elbows and curl the weights while exhaling.

- Continue to raise the weights until your biceps are fully contracted and the dumbbells are at shoulder level.

- Lower the dumbbells while inhaling to the starting position. This exercise targets the biceps.

2. Push-Up:

- Start in a plank position with your hands shoulder-width apart.

- Lower your body by bending your elbows until your chest is close to the ground.

- Push your body back up to the starting position. This exercise targets the chest, shoulders, and triceps.

3. Bent-Over Row:

- Stand with a dumbbell in each hand, palms facing your body.

- Bend your knees slightly and bend at the waist.

- Keep your back straight, and let the dumbbells hang at arm's length.

- Pull the dumbbells to your lower ribcage while keeping your elbows close to your body.

- Lower the dumbbells back to the starting position. This exercise targets the back and biceps.

4. Tricep Dip:

- Sit on a stable surface (e.g., a bench) with your hands placed next to your hips.

- Lift your body off the surface, supporting your weight with your hands.

- Bend your elbows to lower your body and then straighten

them to raise it back up. This exercise targets the triceps.

5. Pull-Up:

- Hang from a pull-up bar with your palms facing away from your body.

- Pull your body up until your chin is above the bar.

- Lower your body back to the starting position. This exercise targets the back and biceps.

5.2 Isotonic Exercises for Lower Body

1. Squats:

- Stand with your feet hip-width apart.

- Bend your knees and hips to lower your body as if sitting back into a chair.

- Keep your back straight and your knees aligned with your toes.

- Return to the standing position. Squats target the quadriceps, hamstrings, and glutes.

2. Lunges:

- Stand with your feet together.

- Step one foot forward and lower your body until both knees are at a 90-degree angle.

- Push off the front foot to return to the starting position.

- Alternate legs for each repetition. Lunges target the

quadriceps, hamstrings, and glutes.

3. Deadlift:

- Stand with a barbell in front of you, feet hip-width apart.

- Bend at your hips and knees to lower your body and grasp the bar with an overhand grip.

- Keep your back straight as you lift the barbell by straightening your hips and knees.

- Lower the barbell back to the ground. Deadlifts target the lower back, glutes, hamstrings, and lower body.

4. Leg Press:

- Sit in a leg press machine with your feet shoulder-width apart.

- Push the weight upwards by
  extending your knees.

- Lower the weight by bending
  your knees. Leg presses target
  the quadriceps, hamstrings, and
  glutes.

5. Calf Raises:

- Stand with the balls of your feet
  on an elevated surface (e.g., a
  step).

- Raise your heels as high as
  possible by extending your
  ankles.

- Lower your heels below the
  step to stretch your calf
  muscles.

- This exercise primarily targets
  the calf muscles.

These isotonic exercises can be incorporated into your workout routine to target specific muscle groups in the upper and lower body, helping you build strength and endurance. Always remember to use proper form and technique to maximize the benefits and minimize the risk of injury.

5.3 Isotonic Exercises for Core

1. Plank:

- Start in a push-up position with your hands directly under your shoulders.

- Keep your body in a straight line from head to heels, engaging your core muscles.

- Hold this position for as long as you can, making sure to breathe steadily. You can start with shorter durations and gradually increase the time as your core strength improves.

2. Russian Twists:

- Sit on the floor with your knees bent and your feet flat.

- Lean back slightly, keeping your back straight, and lift your feet off the ground.

- Hold a weight or a medicine ball in both hands.

- Twist your torso to the right, bringing the weight or ball beside your right hip.

- Return to the center and then twist to the left.

- Continue this twisting motion for the desired number of repetitions.

3. Bicycle Crunches:

- Lie on your back with your hands behind your head and your knees bent.

- Lift your head, shoulders, and feet off the ground.

- Begin by bringing your right elbow and left knee toward each other while extending your right leg.

- Alternate sides in a pedaling motion, bringing your left elbow to your right knee and extending your left leg.

- Continue this motion for the desired number of repetitions.

4. Leg Raises:

- Lie on your back with your hands under your hips or at your sides.

- Keep your legs straight and lift them off the ground to create a 90-degree angle with your upper body.

- Lower your legs back down but don't let them touch the ground before raising them again.

- This exercise targets the lower abdominal muscles.

5. Mountain Climbers:

- Start in a plank position with your hands directly under your shoulders.

- Alternate bringing your knees toward your chest, as if you were running in place.

- Maintain a brisk pace while keeping your core engaged.

- This exercise not only works the core but also provides a cardiovascular challenge.

6. Superman (or Superwoman):

- Lie face down on the ground with your arms extended in front of you.

- Simultaneously lift your arms, chest, and legs off the ground, arching your back.

- Hold this position briefly, then lower back to the ground.

- This exercise targets the lower back and helps improve posture.

7. Stability Ball Rollout:

- Kneel with your hands on a stability ball, arms extended.

- Slowly roll the ball forward, extending your arms, and then roll it back in.

- The goal is to maintain a straight line from your knees to your head during the exercise.

- This exercise challenges both your core and stability.

Incorporate these isotonic core exercises into your routine to build a strong and stable core. A strong core not only improves your posture and helps prevent lower back pain but also enhances overall athletic performance

and daily functional movements.
Always prioritize proper form and
technique to maximize the benefits
and reduce the risk of injury.

CHAPTER 6

Isotonic Exercise vs. Isometric Exercise

6.1 Key Differences

Isotonic Exercise:

- **Muscle Length Change:** Isotonic exercises involve muscle contractions where the length of the muscle changes as it generates force to move a joint through a range of motion.

- **Dynamic Movements:** These exercises are characterized by dynamic movements, such as lifting, pushing, or pulling a resistance.

- **Examples:** Bicep curls, squats, push-ups, and lunges are examples of isotonic exercises.

- **Benefits:** Isotonic exercises are effective for building muscle strength, endurance, and flexibility. They often mimic functional movements and are suitable for overall fitness and sports performance.

Isometric Exercise:

- **Muscle Length Stays the Same:** Isometric exercises involve muscle contractions where the length of the muscle remains constant while generating force. There is no movement at the joint during an isometric contraction.

- **Static Poses:** These exercises are characterized by holding a specific position or posture without joint movement.

- **Examples:** Planks, wall sits, and static wall push-ups are examples of isometric exercises.

- **Benefits:** Isometric exercises help improve muscle endurance, stability, and joint strength. They can be beneficial for rehabilitation, injury prevention, and building strength in specific joint angles.

6.2 When to Choose Isotonic vs. Isometric

Choose Isotonic Exercises When:

- You want to work on muscle strength, size, and endurance.

- You prefer exercises that involve dynamic movements and range of motion.

- You aim to improve overall functional fitness and athletic performance.

- You're looking to target specific muscle groups for development.

- You want to engage in a more traditional workout routine that includes lifting weights or performing bodyweight exercises.

Choose Isometric Exercises When:

- You need to strengthen muscles and joints in a specific position or angle, such as rehabilitation from an injury.

- You want to enhance muscle endurance, stability, and control without joint movement.

- You have limitations in joint mobility that prevent full-range isotonic exercises.

- You seek to improve posture and core stability.

- You prefer exercises that require minimal equipment and can be done anywhere.

In many cases, a balanced fitness routine incorporates both isotonic and isometric exercises. For example, an athlete may use isotonic exercises to build strength and power while incorporating isometric exercises to enhance joint stability and injury prevention. The choice between the two depends on your individual fitness goals, your current physical condition, and the specific benefits you aim to achieve.

CHAPTER 7

Common Mistakes and Tips

7.1 Avoiding Overtraining

Common Mistakes:

1. **Neglecting Rest Days:** One of the most common mistakes is not allowing your body sufficient time to recover. Overtraining often occurs when you don't incorporate rest days into your routine.

2. **Excessive Frequency:** Training the same muscle groups too frequently can lead to overtraining. It's important to

give your muscles time to repair and grow between workouts.

3. **Ignoring Signs of Overtraining:** Many individuals push through fatigue, soreness, and decreased performance, thinking it will lead to faster progress. This can result in overtraining and potential injuries.

4. **Inadequate Sleep and Nutrition:** Not getting enough sleep or proper nutrition can contribute to overtraining. Both sleep and nutrition are essential for recovery and muscle repair.

Tips to Avoid Overtraining:

1. **Include Rest Days:** Plan rest days into your exercise routine to allow your muscles and

central nervous system to recover. Rest days are essential for preventing overtraining.

2. **Vary Your Routine:** Incorporate variety into your workouts to avoid overusing the same muscle groups. This can be achieved by alternating muscle groups worked each day or by changing exercise modalities.

3. **Listen to Your Body:** Pay attention to your body's signals. If you experience extreme fatigue, persistent soreness, or a noticeable decrease in performance, it's a sign that you might be overtraining. Adjust your workout intensity or take additional rest days as needed.

4. **Proper Nutrition:** Ensure you are getting an adequate intake of nutrients, including protein, carbohydrates, and healthy fats, to support your exercise routine. Hydration is also crucial for muscle function and recovery.

5. **Adequate Sleep:** Prioritize sleep and aim for 7-9 hours per night. Sleep is when your body repairs and regenerates, making it a crucial component of recovery.

6. **Periodization:** Consider periodizing your training program, which involves planned variations in intensity and volume over time. This allows for more focused recovery periods.

7. **Use Active Recovery:** On rest days, engage in active recovery activities like light yoga, walking, or swimming. These activities can help promote circulation and reduce muscle soreness.

8. **Monitor Progress:** Keep a training log to track your progress and how you feel during workouts. This can help you identify trends of overtraining and make adjustments as needed.

9. **Consult a Professional:** If you suspect you are overtraining or are experiencing persistent fatigue, it's a good idea to consult a fitness professional or healthcare provider for guidance and potential adjustments to your routine.

By avoiding overtraining and prioritizing proper recovery, you can maintain a sustainable and effective exercise routine that supports your fitness goals while reducing the risk of burnout and injury.

7.2 Setting Realistic Goals

Common Mistakes:

1. **Setting Unrealistic Expectations:** One of the most common mistakes is setting goals that are too ambitious or unrealistic. For example, aiming to lose a significant amount of weight in a very short period can be unrealistic and demotivating.

2. **Focusing Solely on Outcomes:**
Another mistake is solely
focusing on the end result, such
as reaching a specific weight or
body fat percentage, without
considering the process and
intermediate milestones.

3. **Comparing Yourself to
Others:** Comparing your
progress to that of others can
lead to unrealistic goals and
frustration. Everyone's fitness
journey is unique, and
individual progress varies.

4. **Neglecting Smaller Goals:**
Setting only large, long-term
goals without breaking them
down into smaller, more
achievable milestones can make
your journey seem
overwhelming.

Tips for Setting Realistic Goals:

1. **Specificity:** Define your goals with precision. Rather than a vague goal like "getting in shape," set a specific target, such as "losing 10 pounds in three months" or "increasing my bench press by 20 pounds."

2. **Measurability:** Ensure that your goals are measurable and quantifiable. You should be able to track your progress and know when you've achieved your goal.

3. **Achievability:** Consider your current fitness level, lifestyle, and commitments. Your goals should be challenging but realistic. Assess whether you have the time and resources to work towards them.

4. **Relevance:** Ensure that your goals align with your personal values and what's important to you. They should be meaningful and relevant to your life.

5. **Time-Bound:** Set a timeframe for achieving your goals. This adds a sense of urgency and helps you stay accountable. For example, "I will run a 5K race in three months."

6. **Break Goals Down:** Divide larger, long-term goals into smaller, short-term objectives. These interim goals make your progress more manageable and provide a sense of achievement along the way.

7. **Focus on Process Goals:** Instead of solely focusing on

outcomes like weight loss, emphasize process goals. These are actions and behaviors within your control, such as "I will exercise for 30 minutes, five days a week" or "I will eat a serving of vegetables with every meal."

8. **Seek Professional Guidance:** If you're unsure about setting realistic fitness goals, consider consulting a fitness professional or a personal trainer. They can help you develop goals that align with your abilities and needs.

9. **Celebrate Achievements:** Acknowledge and celebrate your achievements, no matter how small they may seem. Recognizing progress and effort can help keep you motivated.

10. **Adjust as Needed:** Be flexible with your goals. If circumstances change or you encounter unexpected challenges, don't be afraid to adjust your goals to stay on track.

Setting realistic goals that are tailored to your abilities and lifestyle, you increase the likelihood of success and long-term motivation in your fitness journey. Remember that achieving your fitness goals is a marathon, not a sprint, and progress should be sustainable and enjoyable.

7.3 Staying Consistent

Staying consistent in your fitness routine is essential for long-term success. Here are common challenges and tips to help you maintain consistency in your exercise regimen:

Common Challenges:

1. **Lack of Motivation:** Staying motivated can be challenging, especially when results are not immediate. Many people struggle with maintaining enthusiasm for their fitness routine.

2. **Busy Schedules:** Balancing work, family, and other commitments can make it difficult to find time for regular exercise.

3. **Plateaus and Frustration:** Hitting a plateau or not seeing the progress you expected can be discouraging and lead to a lack of consistency.

4. **Injury and Overtraining:**
   Injuries or overtraining can
   disrupt your routine and make
   it challenging to stay
   consistent.

Tips for Staying Consistent:

1. **Set Realistic Goals:** As
   mentioned earlier, set
   achievable and realistic fitness
   goals. This can help you
   maintain motivation as you see
   progress.

2. **Create a Routine:** Establish a
   consistent workout schedule.
   Treat exercise like an
   appointment and prioritize it as
   part of your daily or weekly
   routine.

3. **Find Enjoyable Activities:**
   Choose exercises and activities
   that you enjoy. If you like what

you're doing, you're more likely to stick with it.

4. **Mix It Up:** Variety can help keep your routine interesting. Incorporate different types of exercises and activities to prevent boredom.

5. **Accountability:** Find an accountability partner, such as a workout buddy or a fitness app, to help you stay on track.

6. **Small Steps:** If you're struggling with motivation, start with small, manageable changes in your routine. Gradually increase the intensity and duration as your motivation builds.

7. **Visualize Your Goals:** Regularly visualize your fitness goals to keep them at the

forefront of your mind. This
can help maintain motivation.

8. **Celebrate Milestones:**
Celebrate your achievements
and milestones, even if they are
small. This positive
reinforcement can keep you
motivated.

9. **Adapt to Life Changes:** Be
flexible and adapt your routine
to accommodate life changes. If
your schedule or circumstances
change, find ways to continue
your fitness journey.

10. **Mindset:** Develop a positive
mindset. Instead of viewing
exercise as a chore, reframe it
as an opportunity to improve
your health and well-being.

11. **Progress Tracking:** Keep a
record of your workouts, noting

your achievements and areas
where you can improve. This
can help you see how far you've
come.

12. **Recovery:** Don't underestimate
the importance of rest and
recovery. It's an essential part
of staying consistent and
preventing burnout.

13. **Seek Support:** If you're
struggling with consistency,
consider seeking support from a
fitness professional or a
therapist who specializes in
behavior change.

consistency is key to achieving and
maintaining your fitness goals. It's
normal to have periods of lower
motivation or temporary setbacks, but
by implementing these tips and
strategies, you can increase your

chances of staying on course with your fitness journey.

7.4 Emphasizing Its Role in a Healthy Lifestyle

Emphasizing the role of exercise in a healthy lifestyle is crucial because regular physical activity offers numerous benefits for both physical and mental well-being. Here are some key points to underscore the importance of exercise in a healthy lifestyle:

1. **Physical Health:** Regular exercise is essential for maintaining a healthy body. It helps prevent and manage various health conditions, including cardiovascular

diseases, diabetes, obesity, and certain types of cancer.

2. **Weight Management:** Exercise plays a significant role in managing body weight. It helps with both weight loss and weight maintenance by burning calories and increasing metabolic rate.

3. **Muscle and Bone Health:** Engaging in weight-bearing and resistance exercises promotes muscle strength and bone density. This is particularly important for aging adults in preventing osteoporosis and frailty.

4. **Improved Cardiovascular Health:** Exercise strengthens the heart and circulatory system, reducing the risk of

heart disease. It can help lower blood pressure, improve cholesterol levels, and enhance overall cardiovascular health.

5. **Mental Well-Being:** Regular physical activity is associated with reduced symptoms of depression and anxiety. It also promotes the release of endorphins, which are natural mood enhancers.

6. **Stress Reduction:** Exercise is an effective stress reliever. It helps manage the body's response to stress, reducing tension and anxiety.

7. **Quality Sleep:** A healthy lifestyle includes regular and quality sleep. Exercise can improve sleep patterns and help with insomnia.

8. **Enhanced Cognitive Function:** Physical activity has a positive impact on cognitive function, memory, and mental clarity. It can reduce the risk of cognitive decline and improve overall brain health.

9. **Energy and Productivity:** Regular exercise boosts energy levels and can enhance daily productivity. It can help you feel more alert and focused throughout the day.

10. **Social Interaction:** Many forms of exercise, such as team sports or group fitness classes, provide opportunities for social interaction and the development of a support network.

11. **Healthy Habits:** Incorporating exercise into your daily routine

often leads to the adoption of other healthy habits, including balanced nutrition, hydration, and stress management.

12. **Longevity:** Studies have shown that regular physical activity is associated with a longer life and reduced mortality from various causes.

13. **Prevention of Lifestyle Diseases:** Exercise is a primary component of preventing lifestyle-related diseases. It complements a balanced diet and a non-sedentary lifestyle to promote overall health.

14. **Personal Growth and Achievement:** Achieving fitness goals and milestones through exercise fosters a sense

of personal accomplishment and self-esteem.

15. **Inspiration and Role Modeling:** Leading a healthy, active lifestyle can inspire others to do the same, creating a positive ripple effect within families and communities.

Emphasizing the central role of exercise in a healthy lifestyle, individuals are more likely to prioritize physical activity, recognize its numerous benefits, and make it a regular part of their lives. Regular exercise not only enhances physical health but also contributes to mental and emotional well-being, leading to a holistic approach to overall health and vitality.

www.ingramcontent.com/pod-product-compliance
Lightning Source LLC
Chambersburg PA
CBHW070822280726
48660CB00017B/2399